CANNABIS COOKBOOK

3

CANNABIS COOKBOOK

TABLE OF CONTENTS

Ice Creams and Sorbets:

Cannabis Vanilla Ice Cream p.81

Cannabis Lemon Sorbet p.82

Cannabis Berry Popsicle p.83

Street Food:

Cannabis Cheese Pretzels with Sauce p.85

Cannabis Guacamole Nachos p.86

Cannabis Caramelized Onion Hot Dog p.87

Light Dishes:

Cannabis Quinoa and Avocado Salad with Dressing p.89

Cannabis Sushi with Soy Sauce p.90

Cannabis Chicken Wrap with Sauce p.91

Mediterranean Cuisine:

Cannabis Hummus with Pita p.93

Cannabis Eggplant Parmesan p.94

Cannabis Asparagus Risotto p.95

Vegan Dishes:

Cannabis Chickpea Burger p.97

Cannabis Vegetable Couscous p.98

Cannabis Tofu Curry p.99

Breakfast Dishes:

Cannabis Pancakes with Maple Syrup p.102

Cannabis Smoothie Bowl p.103

Apple Cannabis Porridge p.104

Autumn Dishes:

Cannabis Stuffed Pumpkin p.106

CANNABIS COOKBOOK

Hey there, fellow flavor enthusiasts!

Get ready for a culinary escapade like no other. This isn't just about cooking; it's about infusing some serious vibes into your kitchen. So, why are we diving into the world of cannabis-infused recipes? Well, it's not just about creating tasty treats; it's about turning your kitchen into a flavor-packed haven with a sprinkle of good vibes.

In the past, cannabis might've been associated with just a laid-back weekend, but times are changing. Cannabis has graduated from being just a recreational sidekick to becoming the rockstar of holistic wellness. Our recipes aren't just about getting a buzz; they're about enhancing your culinary journey and maybe adding a little extra glow to your well-being.

From starters to sweets, each recipe is like a little pot (pun intended) of joy. We're not just cooking; we're creating experiences that excite the taste buds and add a little extra sunshine to your day.

So, what's the deal with cannabis in the kitchen? Well, besides being the life of the party, it brings a whole bunch of feel-good benefits. Think relaxation, stress relief, and a dash of pain management—all served up in a tasty dish.

Whether you're a seasoned cannabis chef or just curious, join us in this adventure where every bite is a high-five to your senses. Let's explore the amazing synergy of cannabis and cuisine, turning every meal into a celebration of life's flavors.

So, grab your apron, get ready to cook up a storm, and let's infuse some good vibes into your kitchen and beyond!

Happy cooking and living your best, high-on-life life!

Appetizers

1. Cannabis Pesto Toasts

Ingredients for 4:

- 4 slices of Tuscan bread
- 2 cups fresh basil leaves
- 1/2 cup pine nuts
- 2 cloves of garlic
- 1/2 cup grated Parmesan cheese
- 1/2 cup extra virgin olive oil
- 1-2 tablespoons cannabis-infused oil (depending on desired potency)
- Salt and pepper to taste

Prep Time: 15 minutes

Instructions:

1. **Crafting the Cannabis Pesto:**

   - Blend fresh basil, pine nuts, garlic, Parmesan, and olive oil in a blender.
   - Blitz the ingredients until they form a creamy consistency.
   - Add cannabis-infused oil to the pesto and mix well. Ensure the dosage is evenly distributed.

2. **Toasting the Bread:**

   - Grill or toast the Tuscan bread slices until they achieve a crispy texture.

3. **Assembling the Toasts:**

   - Generously spread the cannabis pesto on the toasted Tuscan bread slices.

- Season with salt and pepper to taste.

4. **Serving:**

  - Arrange the toasts on a serving plate.

  - Optionally garnish with fresh basil or a light sprinkle of Parmesan.

Nutritional Information (per serving): *(Nutritional values are approximate and may vary based on specific ingredients used.)*

- Calories: 300 kcal

- Protein: 8g

- Fat: 25g

  - Saturated: 5g

  - Monounsaturated: 15g

  - Polyunsaturated: 3g

- Carbohydrates: 10g

  - Sugars: 1g

- Fiber: 2g

2. Cannabis-infused Potato Croquettes

Ingredients for 4:

- 4 large potatoes, peeled and mashed
- 1/2 cup breadcrumbs
- 1/4 cup cannabis-infused olive oil
- 2 tablespoons chopped parsley
- Salt and pepper to taste
- 2 eggs, beaten
- Vegetable oil for frying

Preparation Time: 30 minutes
Cook Time: 15 minutes
Total Time: 45 minutes

Procedure:

1. In a bowl, combine mashed potatoes, breadcrumbs, cannabis-infused olive oil, chopped parsley, salt, and pepper.
2. Shape the mixture into small croquettes.
3. Dip each croquette into beaten eggs.
4. Heat vegetable oil in a pan and fry croquettes until golden brown.
5. Drain excess oil on paper towels.
6. Serve hot and enjoy your cannabis-infused potato croquettes!

Nutritional Information (per serving):

- Calories: 250
- Protein: 5g
- Carbohydrates: 35g
- Fat: 10g
- Fiber: 4g

3. Cannabis Guacamole

Ingredients for 4:

- 3 ripe avocados, mashed
- 1/2 cup diced tomatoes
- 1/4 cup finely chopped red onion
- 2 tablespoons chopped cilantro
- 1 jalapeño, finely chopped (seeds removed for less heat)
- Juice of 2 limes
- Salt and pepper to taste
- 1/4 cup cannabis-infused olive oil

Preparation Time: 15 minutes
Total Time: 15 minutes

Procedure:

1. In a bowl, combine mashed avocados, diced tomatoes, red onion, cilantro, and jalapeño.
2. Squeeze in lime juice, add salt and pepper to taste.
3. Drizzle cannabis-infused olive oil and mix well.
4. Serve with tortilla chips and savor your cannabis-infused guacamole!

Nutritional Information (per serving):

- Calories: 180
- Protein: 2g
- Carbohydrates: 12g
- Fat: 15g
- Fiber: 7g

Soups and Salads

4. Cannabis Tomato Soup

Ingredients for 4:

- 6 large tomatoes, diced
- 1 onion, chopped
- 2 cloves garlic, minced
- 1/4 cup cannabis-infused olive oil
- 4 cups vegetable broth
- Salt and pepper to taste
- Fresh basil leaves for garnish

Preparation Time: 15 minutes
Cook Time: 25 minutes
Total Time: 40 minutes

Procedure:

1. In a pot, sauté onions and garlic in cannabis-infused olive oil until softened.
2. Add diced tomatoes and cook until they release their juices.
3. Pour in vegetable broth and bring to a simmer.
4. Blend the soup until smooth.
5. Season with salt and pepper.
6. Garnish with fresh basil leaves.
7. Serve and relish your cannabis-infused tomato soup!

Nutritional Information (per serving):

- Calories: 150
- Protein: 3g
- Carbohydrates: 20g
- Fat: 8g
- Fiber: 5g

5. Cannabis Quinoa Salad

Ingredients for 4:

- 1 cup quinoa, cooked and cooled
- 1 cucumber, diced
- 1 bell pepper, diced
- 1/2 cup cherry tomatoes, halved
- 1/4 cup feta cheese, crumbled
- 2 tablespoons chopped fresh mint
- 1/4 cup cannabis-infused olive oil
- Juice of 1 lemon
- Salt and pepper to taste

Preparation Time: 20 minutes
Total Time: 20 minutes

Procedure:

1. In a large bowl, combine quinoa, cucumber, bell pepper, cherry tomatoes, feta cheese, and mint.
2. In a small bowl, whisk together cannabis-infused olive oil, lemon juice, salt, and pepper.
3. Pour the dressing over the salad and toss well.
4. Serve chilled and enjoy your cannabis-infused quinoa salad!

Nutritional Information (per serving):

- Calories: 280
- Protein: 8g
- Carbohydrates: 30g
- Fat: 15g
- Fiber: 5g

6. Cannabis Butternut Squash Velouté

Ingredients for 4:

- 2 cups pumpkin puree
- 1 onion, chopped
- 2 cloves garlic, minced
- 1/4 cup cannabis-infused olive oil
- 4 cups vegetable broth
- 1/2 teaspoon ground nutmeg
- Salt and pepper to taste
- 1/2 cup heavy cream (optional)
- Pumpkin seeds for garnish

Preparation Time: 15 minutes
Cook Time: 25 minutes
Total Time: 40 minutes

Procedure:

1. In a pot, sauté onions and garlic in cannabis-infused olive oil until softened.
2. Add pumpkin puree, vegetable broth, nutmeg, salt, and pepper.
3. Simmer until the soup is heated through.
4. Blend until smooth.
5. Stir in heavy cream if desired.
6. Garnish with pumpkin seeds.
7. Serve and enjoy your creamy cannabis-infused pumpkin soup!

Nutritional Information (per serving):

- Calories: 200
- Protein: 3g
- Carbohydrates: 20g
- Fat: 14g
- Fiber: 5g

Main Courses – Pasta

7. Cannabis Pesto Pasta

Ingredients for 4:

- 1 lb (450g) pasta of your choice
- 2 cups fresh basil leaves
- 1/2 cup grated Parmesan cheese
- 1/2 cup cannabis-infused olive oil
- 1/4 cup pine nuts
- 2 cloves garlic, minced
- Salt and pepper to taste

Preparation Time: 15 minutes
Cook Time: 10 minutes
Total Time: 25 minutes

Procedure:

1. Cook pasta according to package instructions.
2. In a food processor, blend basil, Parmesan, cannabis-infused olive oil, pine nuts, garlic, salt, and pepper until smooth.
3. Toss the pesto with the cooked pasta.
4. Serve hot and relish your cannabis-infused pesto pasta!

Nutritional Information (per serving):

- Calories: 450
- Protein: 12g
- Carbohydrates: 40g
- Fat: 25g
- Fiber: 3g

8. Cannabis Ricotta Cannelloni

Ingredients for 4:

- 12 cannelloni tubes, cooked
- 2 cups ricotta cheese
- 1/2 cup grated Parmesan cheese
- 1/4 cup cannabis-infused olive oil
- 2 eggs, beaten
- 2 cups marinara sauce
- Salt and pepper to taste
- Fresh basil leaves for garnish

Preparation Time: 20 minutes
Cook Time: 25 minutes
Total Time: 45 minutes

Procedure:

1. In a bowl, mix ricotta, Parmesan, cannabis-infused olive oil, beaten eggs, salt, and pepper.
2. Stuff the cannelloni tubes with the ricotta mixture.
3. Place stuffed cannelloni in a baking dish and cover with marinara sauce.
4. Bake until bubbly and golden.
5. Garnish with fresh basil leaves.
6. Serve and enjoy your cannabis-infused ricotta cannelloni!

Nutritional Information (per serving):

- Calories: 380
- Protein: 18g
- Carbohydrates: 30g
- Fat: 20g

9. Cannabis Spaghetti Aglio e Olio e Peperoncino

Ingredients for 4:

- 1 lb (450g) spaghetti
- 1/2 cup cannabis-infused olive oil
- 6 cloves garlic, thinly sliced
- Red pepper flakes to taste
- Fresh parsley, chopped
- Grated Parmesan cheese for topping
- Salt and pepper to taste

Preparation Time: 10 minutes
Cook Time: 10 minutes
Total Time: 20 minutes

Procedure:

1. Cook spaghetti according to package instructions.
2. In a pan, heat cannabis-infused olive oil and sauté garlic until golden.
3. Add red pepper flakes, salt, and pepper.
4. Toss cooked spaghetti in the infused oil.
5. Garnish with chopped fresh parsley and grated Parmesan.
6. Serve hot and savor your cannabis-infused Spaghetti Aglio e Olio!

Nutritional Information (per serving):

- Calories: 480
- Protein: 10g
- Carbohydrates: 50g
- Fat: 25g
- Fiber: 3g

Main courses-Meat

10. Cannabis Curry Chicken

Ingredients for 4:

- 4 chicken breasts, diced
- 1 onion, finely chopped
- 2 cloves garlic, minced
- 1/4 cup cannabis-infused coconut oil
- 2 tablespoons curry powder
- 1 can (14 oz) coconut milk
- 1 cup vegetables of choice (bell peppers, peas, carrots)
- Salt and pepper to taste
- Fresh cilantro for garnish

Preparation Time: 20 minutes
Cook Time: 30 minutes
Total Time: 50 minutes

Procedure:

1. In a pan, sauté onions and garlic in cannabis-infused coconut oil until softened.
2. Add diced chicken and cook until browned.
3. Stir in curry powder and cook for an additional 2 minutes.
4. Pour in coconut milk and add vegetables. Simmer until chicken is cooked through.
5. Season with salt and pepper.
6. Garnish with fresh cilantro.
7. Serve over rice and enjoy your cannabis-infused curry chicken!

Nutritional Information (per serving):

- Calories: 400
- Protein: 25g
- Carbohydrates: 15g
- Fat: 30g
- Fiber: 3g

11. Cannabis Chili con Carne

Ingredients for 4:

- 1 lb ground beef
- 1 onion, diced
- 2 cloves garlic, minced
- 1 can (14 oz) kidney beans, drained and rinsed
- 1 can (14 oz) crushed tomatoes
- 1 cup beef broth
- 2 tablespoons chili powder
- 1 teaspoon cumin
- Salt and pepper to taste
- 1/4 cup cannabis-infused olive oil
- Shredded cheddar cheese and green onions for topping

Preparation Time: 20 minutes
Cook Time: 30 minutes
Total Time: 50 minutes

Procedure:

1. In a pot, sauté onions and garlic in cannabis-infused olive oil until softened.
2. Add ground beef and cook until browned.
3. Stir in chili powder, cumin, kidney beans, crushed tomatoes, and beef broth.
4. Simmer for 25-30 minutes.
5. Season with salt and pepper.
6. Top with shredded cheddar cheese and green onions.
7. Serve hot and relish your cannabis-infused chili con carne!

Nutritional Information (per serving):

- Calories: 450
- Protein: 30g
- Carbohydrates: 25g
- Fat: 25g
- Fiber: 6g

12. Glazed Cannabis Pork Tenderloin

Ingredients for 4:

- 2 pork tenderloins
- 1/2 cup soy sauce
- 1/4 cup honey
- 2 tablespoons cannabis-infused olive oil
- 2 cloves garlic, minced
- 1 teaspoon ginger, grated
- Salt and pepper to taste
- Sesame seeds and chopped green onions for garnish

Preparation Time: 15 minutes
Cook Time: 25 minutes
Total Time: 40 minutes

Procedure:

1. Preheat oven to 375°F (190°C).
2. Season pork tenderloins with salt and pepper.
3. In a bowl, mix soy sauce, honey, cannabis-infused olive oil, garlic, and ginger.
4. Brush the glaze over the pork.
5. Roast in the oven for 25 minutes or until cooked through.
6. Garnish with sesame seeds and chopped green onions.
7. Slice and serve your glazed cannabis-infused pork tenderloin!

Nutritional Information (per serving):

- Calories: 350
- Protein: 30g
- Carbohydrates: 20g
- Fat: 15g
- Fiber: 1g

Main Courses – Fish:

13. Grilled Salmon with Cannabis Sauce

Ingredients for 4:

- 4 salmon fillets
- 1/4 cup cannabis-infused olive oil
- 2 tablespoons soy sauce
- 1 tablespoon Dijon mustard
- 1 tablespoon honey
- 2 cloves garlic, minced
- Lemon wedges for serving
- Fresh dill for garnish

Preparation Time: 15 minutes
Cook Time: 10 minutes
Total Time: 25 minutes

Procedure:

1. Preheat the grill to medium-high heat.
2. In a bowl, whisk together cannabis-infused olive oil, soy sauce, Dijon mustard, honey, and minced garlic.
3. Brush the salmon fillets with the marinade.
4. Grill the salmon for 4-5 minutes per side or until cooked through.
5. Drizzle with extra marinade before serving.
6. Garnish with fresh dill and serve with lemon wedges.
7. Enjoy your grilled cannabis-infused salmon!

Nutritional Information (per serving):

- Calories: 300
- Protein: 25g
- Carbohydrates: 5g
- Fat: 20g
- Fiber: 1g

14. Cannabis Seafood Risotto

Ingredients for 4:

- 1 cup Arborio rice
- 1/2 cup dry white wine
- 4 cups seafood broth
- 1 lb mixed seafood (shrimp, mussels, calamari)
- 1/4 cup cannabis-infused olive oil
- 1 onion, finely chopped
- 2 cloves garlic, minced
- 1/2 cup grated Parmesan cheese
- Fresh parsley for garnish
- Salt and pepper to taste

Preparation Time: 15 minutes
Cook Time: 25 minutes
Total Time: 40 minutes

Procedure:

1. In a pan, sauté onions and garlic in cannabis-infused olive oil until softened.
2. Add Arborio rice and cook until translucent.
3. Pour in white wine and let it evaporate.
4. Gradually add seafood broth, stirring constantly until the rice is cooked.
5. In a separate pan, cook mixed seafood in cannabis-infused olive oil until done.
6. Stir seafood and Parmesan into the risotto.
7. Season with salt and pepper.
8. Garnish with fresh parsley.

9. Serve hot and enjoy your cannabis-infused seafood risotto!

Nutritional Information (per serving):

- Calories: 450
- Protein: 25g
- Carbohydrates: 50g
- Fat: 18g
- Fiber: 2g

15. Spicy Cannabis Shrimp

Ingredients for 4:

- 1 lb large shrimp, peeled and deveined
- 1/4 cup cannabis-infused olive oil
- 2 cloves garlic, minced
- 1 teaspoon smoked paprika
- 1/2 teaspoon cayenne pepper
- Salt and pepper to taste
- Fresh lemon wedges for serving
- Chopped parsley for garnish

Preparation Time: 10 minutes
Cook Time: 5 minutes
Total Time: 15 minutes

Procedure:

1. In a pan, heat cannabis-infused olive oil over medium heat.
2. Add minced garlic and cook until fragrant.
3. Add shrimp, smoked paprika, cayenne pepper, salt, and pepper.
4. Cook for 2-3 minutes per side or until shrimp are opaque.
5. Serve with fresh lemon wedges and garnish with chopped parsley.
6. Enjoy your spicy cannabis-infused shrimp!

Nutritional Information (per serving):

- Calories: 220
- Protein: 20g
- Carbohydrates: 2g
- Fat: 15g
- Fiber: 0g

Sides

16. Cannabis Rosemary Roasted Potatoes

Ingredients for 4:

- 4 large potatoes, diced
- 1/4 cup cannabis-infused olive oil
- 1 tablespoon fresh rosemary, chopped
- Salt and pepper to taste

Preparation Time: 10 minutes
Cook Time: 30 minutes
Total Time: 40 minutes

Procedure:

1. Preheat the oven to 400°F (200°C).
2. In a bowl, toss diced potatoes with cannabis-infused olive oil, chopped rosemary, salt, and pepper.
3. Spread the potatoes on a baking sheet in a single layer.
4. Roast for 25-30 minutes or until golden brown and crispy.
5. Serve hot and relish your cannabis-infused roasted rosemary potatoes!

Nutritional Information (per serving):

- Calories: 180
- Protein: 3g
- Carbohydrates: 30g
- Fat: 7g
- Fiber: 3g

17. Cannabis Potato Salad

Ingredients for 4:

- 4 large potatoes, boiled and diced
- 1/2 cup mayonnaise
- 2 tablespoons Dijon mustard
- 1/4 cup cannabis-infused olive oil
- 1/4 cup chopped dill pickles
- 2 tablespoons chopped fresh parsley
- Salt and pepper to taste
- Hard-boiled eggs for garnish

Preparation Time: 20 minutes
Total Time: 20 minutes

Procedure:

1. In a large bowl, combine diced potatoes, mayonnaise, Dijon mustard, cannabis-infused olive oil, dill pickles, parsley, salt, and pepper.
2. Mix until well combined.
3. Garnish with slices of hard-boiled eggs.
4. Chill before serving.
5. Enjoy your cannabis-infused potato salad!

Nutritional Information (per serving):

- Calories: 250
- Protein: 4g
- Carbohydrates: 25g
- Fat: 15g
- Fiber: 3g

18. Grilled Vegetables with Cannabis Marinade
Ingredients for 4:

- 2 zucchinis, sliced
- 1 eggplant, sliced
- 1 bell pepper, sliced
- 1 red onion, sliced
- 1/4 cup cannabis-infused olive oil
- 2 tablespoons balsamic vinegar
- 2 cloves garlic, minced
- 1 teaspoon Italian seasoning
- Salt and pepper to taste
- Fresh basil for garnish

Preparation Time: 15 minutes
Cook Time: 10 minutes
Total Time: 25 minutes

Procedure:

1. In a bowl, whisk together cannabis-infused olive oil, balsamic vinegar, minced garlic, Italian seasoning, salt, and pepper.
2. Toss sliced vegetables in the marinade until well coated.
3. Grill the vegetables until tender and slightly charred.
4. Garnish with fresh basil.
5. Serve and relish your cannabis-infused grilled marinated vegetables!

Nutritional Information (per serving):

- Calories: 180
- Protein: 3g
- Carbohydrates: 20g
- Fat: 10g
- Fiber: 5g

Sandwiches and Wraps

19. Cannabis Chicken Mayo Sandwich

Ingredients for 4

- 2 cups shredded cooked chicken
- 1/2 cup mayonnaise
- 1/4 cup cannabis-infused olive oil
- 2 tablespoons Dijon mustard
- 1 celery stalk, finely chopped
- Salt and pepper to taste
- Lettuce leaves
- Bread slices for serving

Preparation Time: 15 minutes
Total Time: 15 minutes

Procedure:

1. In a bowl, combine shredded chicken, mayonnaise, cannabis-infused olive oil, Dijon mustard, and chopped celery.
2. Mix until well combined.
3. Season with salt and pepper to taste.
4. Spread the chicken mayo mixture on bread slices.
5. Top with lettuce leaves.
6. Assemble sandwiches and enjoy your cannabis-infused chicken mayo sandwich!

Nutritional Information (per serving):

- Calories: 350
- Protein: 15g
- Carbohydrates: 20g
- Fat: 25g
- Fiber: 2g

20. Cannabis Club Sandwich

Ingredients for 4:

- 8 slices bread
- 1/2 cup cannabis-infused mayonnaise
- 8 slices cooked bacon
- 2 cooked chicken breasts, sliced
- Lettuce leaves
- Tomato slices
- Salt and pepper to taste

Preparation Time: 15 minutes
Total Time: 15 minutes

Procedure:

1. Toast the bread slices.
2. Spread cannabis-infused mayonnaise on one side of each slice.
3. Layer bacon, sliced chicken, lettuce, and tomato on half of the bread slices.
4. Season with salt and pepper to taste.
5. Top with the remaining slices to create sandwiches.
6. Secure with toothpicks if needed.
7. Slice in half and enjoy your cannabis-infused club sandwich!

Nutritional Information (per serving):

- Calories: 450
- Protein: 20g
- Carbohydrates: 30g
- Fat: 25g
- Fiber: 3g

21. Caprese Sanwich Panini with Cannabis Pesto

Ingredients for 4:

- 8 slices ciabatta or Italian bread
- 1/2 cup cannabis-infused pesto
- 2 large tomatoes, sliced
- 1 lb fresh mozzarella, sliced
- Fresh basil leaves
- 1/4 cup cannabis-infused olive oil

Preparation Time: 15 minutes
Cook Time: 10 minutes
Total Time: 25 minutes

Procedure:

1. Preheat a panini press or grill pan.
2. Spread cannabis-infused pesto on one side of each bread slice.
3. Layer tomato slices, mozzarella, and fresh basil on half of the slices.
4. Top with the remaining bread slices to create sandwiches.
5. Brush the outsides of the sandwiches with cannabis-infused olive oil.
6. Grill until the cheese is melted and the bread is golden brown.
7. Slice and enjoy your cannabis-infused Caprese panini!

Nutritional Information (per serving):

- Calories: 400
- Protein: 15g
- Carbohydrates: 30g
- Fat: 25g
- Fiber: 2g

Pizza and Focaccia

22. Cannabis Margherita Pizza

Ingredients for 4:

- 1 lb pizza dough
- 1/2 cup cannabis-infused tomato sauce
- 8 oz fresh mozzarella, sliced
- Fresh basil leaves
- 1/4 cup cannabis-infused olive oil
- Salt and pepper to taste

Preparation Time: 15 minutes
Cook Time: 15 minutes
Total Time: 30 minutes

Procedure:

1. Preheat the oven to the highest temperature (usually around 475°F or 245°C).
2. Roll out the pizza dough on a floured surface.
3. Transfer the dough to a pizza stone or baking sheet.
4. Spread cannabis-infused tomato sauce evenly over the dough.
5. Arrange fresh mozzarella slices on top.
6. Season with salt and pepper to taste.
7. Drizzle cannabis-infused olive oil over the pizza.
8. Bake until the crust is golden and the cheese is bubbly (about 12-15 minutes).
9. Top with fresh basil leaves.
10. Slice and savor your cannabis-infused Margherita pizza!

Nutritional Information (per serving):

- Calories: 400
- Protein: 15g
- Carbohydrates: 40g
- Fat: 20g
- Fiber: 2g

23. Cannabis Garlic Focaccia

Ingredients for 4:

- 1 lb pizza dough
- 1/4 cup cannabis-infused olive oil
- 3 cloves garlic, minced
- Fresh rosemary, chopped
- Coarse salt for sprinkling

Preparation Time: 15 minutes
Cook Time: 15 minutes
Total Time: 30 minutes

Procedure:

1. Preheat the oven to 475°F (245°C).
2. Roll out the pizza dough on a floured surface.
3. Transfer the dough to a baking sheet.
4. In a small bowl, mix cannabis-infused olive oil and minced garlic.
5. Brush the dough with the garlic-infused olive oil mixture.
6. Sprinkle with fresh rosemary and coarse salt.
7. Bake until golden and crisp (about 12-15 minutes).
8. Slice and enjoy your cannabis-infused garlic focaccia!

Nutritional Information (per serving):

- Calories: 300
- Protein: 8g
- Carbohydrates: 40g
- Fat: 15g
- Fiber: 2g

24. Cannabis Stuffed Calzone

Ingredients for 4:

- 1 lb pizza dough
- 1/2 cup cannabis-infused tomato sauce
- 1/2 lb Italian sausage, cooked and crumbled
- 1 cup ricotta cheese
- 1 cup shredded mozzarella
- 1/4 cup grated Parmesan
- 1 egg, beaten
- Fresh basil for garnish

Preparation Time: 15 minutes
Cook Time: 20 minutes
Total Time: 35 minutes

Procedure:

1. Preheat the oven to 475°F (245°C).
2. Roll out the pizza dough on a floured surface.
3. Transfer the dough to a pizza stone or baking sheet.
4. Spread cannabis-infused tomato sauce over half of the dough.
5. Layer cooked sausage, ricotta, mozzarella, and Parmesan on one side.
6. Fold the other half of the dough over the filling and seal the edges.
7. Brush the calzone with beaten egg.
8. Bake until golden and crispy (about 18-20 minutes).
9. Garnish with fresh basil.
10. Slice and enjoy your cannabis-infused stuffed calzone!

Nutritional Information (per serving):

- Calories: 450
- Protein: 20g
- Carbohydrates: 40g
- Fat: 25g
- Fiber: 2g

International Dishes

25. Cannabis Carnitas Tacos

Ingredients for 4:

- 1 lb pork shoulder, diced
- 1 onion, sliced
- 3 cloves garlic, minced
- 1/4 cup cannabis-infused olive oil
- 1 teaspoon cumin
- 1 teaspoon smoked paprika
- 1/2 teaspoon chili powder
- Salt and pepper to taste
- Corn tortillas
- Fresh cilantro and diced onions for topping

Preparation Time: 20 minutes
Cook Time: 2 hours
Total Time: 2 hours 20 minutes

Procedure:

1. Preheat the oven to 325°F (163°C).
2. In an oven-safe pot, heat cannabis-infused olive oil.
3. Sear pork shoulder until browned on all sides.
4. Add sliced onions, minced garlic, cumin, smoked paprika, chili powder, salt, and pepper.
5. Cover and transfer to the oven.
6. Cook for 2 hours or until pork is tender.
7. Shred the pork with a fork.
8. Warm corn tortillas and fill with carnitas.
9. Top with fresh cilantro and diced onions.

10.Enjoy your cannabis-infused carnitas tacos!

Nutritional Information (per serving):

- Calories: 350
- Protein: 20g
- Carbohydrates: 20g
- Fat: 20g
- Fiber: 3g

26. Cannabis Lamb Curry

Ingredients for 4:

- 1 lb lamb, diced
- 1 onion, finely chopped
- 2 cloves garlic, minced
- 1/4 cup cannabis-infused coconut oil
- 1 tablespoon curry powder
- 1 can (14 oz) coconut milk
- 1 cup vegetables of choice (peas, carrots, potatoes)
- Salt and pepper to taste
- Fresh cilantro for garnish
- Cooked rice for serving

Preparation Time: 20 minutes
Cook Time: 30 minutes
Total Time: 50 minutes

Procedure:

1. In a pot, sauté onions and garlic in cannabis-infused coconut oil until softened.
2. Add diced lamb and cook until browned.
3. Stir in curry powder and cook for an additional 2 minutes.
4. Pour in coconut milk and add vegetables. Simmer until lamb is cooked through.
5. Season with salt and pepper.
6. Garnish with fresh cilantro.
7. Serve over cooked rice and enjoy your cannabis-infused lamb curry!

Nutritional Information (per serving):

- Calories: 450
- Protein: 25g
- Carbohydrates: 20g
- Fat: 30g
- Fiber: 3g

27. Cannabis Ramen

Ingredients for 4:

- 4 packs ramen noodles
- 1/4 cup cannabis-infused sesame oil
- 2 cloves garlic, minced
- 1 tablespoon ginger, grated
- 1/4 cup soy sauce
- 1 tablespoon miso paste
- 4 cups vegetable broth
- Toppings: sliced green onions, mushrooms, soft-boiled eggs

Preparation Time: 15 minutes
Cook Time: 15 minutes
Total Time: 30 minutes

Procedure:

1. Cook ramen noodles according to package instructions.
2. In a pot, heat cannabis-infused sesame oil and sauté garlic and ginger until fragrant.
3. Add soy sauce, miso paste, and vegetable broth. Bring to a simmer.
4. Divide cooked ramen noodles among bowls.
5. Pour hot broth over the noodles.
6. Top with sliced green onions, mushrooms, and soft-boiled eggs.
7. Serve and savor your cannabis-infused ramen!

Nutritional Information (per serving):

- Calories: 350
- Protein: 10g
- Carbohydrates: 40g
- Fat: 15g
- Fiber: 3g

Desserts

28. Cannabis Brownies

Ingredients for 4:

- 1/2 cup cannabis-infused butter, melted
- 1 cup granulated sugar
- 2 large eggs
- 1 teaspoon vanilla extract
- 1/3 cup cocoa powder
- 1/2 cup all-purpose flour
- 1/4 teaspoon baking powder
- 1/4 teaspoon salt
- 1/2 cup chopped nuts (optional)

Preparation Time: 15 minutes
Cook Time: 25 minutes
Total Time: 40 minutes

Procedure:

1. Preheat the oven to 350°F (175°C).
2. In a bowl, combine melted cannabis-infused butter and sugar.
3. Beat in eggs and vanilla extract until well combined.
4. In a separate bowl, whisk together cocoa powder, flour, baking powder, and salt.
5. Gradually add the dry ingredients to the wet ingredients, mixing until smooth.
6. Fold in chopped nuts if desired.
7. Pour the batter into a greased baking pan.
8. Bake for 20-25 minutes or until a toothpick inserted comes out with moist crumbs.

9. Allow to cool before cutting into squares.

10.Enjoy your cannabis-infused brownies!

Nutritional Information (per serving):

- Calories: 250
- Protein: 4g
- Carbohydrates: 30g
- Fat: 15g
- Fiber: 2g

29. Cannabis Tiramisu

Ingredients for 4:

- 1 cup strong brewed coffee, cooled
- 1/4 cup cannabis-infused coffee liqueur
- 3 large egg yolks
- 1/2 cup granulated sugar
- 1 cup mascarpone cheese
- 1 cup heavy cream
- 24 ladyfinger cookies
- Cocoa powder for dusting

Preparation Time: 30 minutes
Chill Time: 4 hours
Total Time: 4 hours 30 minutes

Procedure:

1. In a bowl, combine brewed coffee and cannabis-infused coffee liqueur. Set aside.
2. In another bowl, whisk together egg yolks and sugar until pale and creamy.
3. Add mascarpone cheese and mix until smooth.
4. In a separate bowl, whip the heavy cream until stiff peaks form.
5. Gently fold the whipped cream into the mascarpone mixture.
6. Dip ladyfingers into the coffee mixture and arrange a layer in a serving dish.
7. Spread half of the mascarpone mixture over the ladyfingers.
8. Repeat the layers with the remaining ladyfingers and mascarpone mixture.

9. Dust the top with cocoa powder.

10. Refrigerate for at least 4 hours before serving.

11. Enjoy your cannabis-infused tiramisu!

Nutritional Information (per serving):

- Calories: 400

- Protein: 6g

- Carbohydrates: 30g

- Fat: 30g

- Fiber: 1g

30. Cannabis Chocolate Chip Muffins

Ingredients for 4:

- 2 cups all-purpose flour
- 1/2 cup sugar
- 1 tablespoon baking powder
- 1/2 teaspoon salt
- 1 cup milk
- 1/4 cup cannabis-infused vegetable oil
- 1 large egg
- 1 teaspoon vanilla extract
- 1/2 cup chocolate chips

Preparation Time: 15 minutes
Bake Time: 20 minutes
Total Time: 35 minutes

Procedure:

1. Preheat the oven to 375°F (190°C). Line a muffin tin with paper liners.
2. In a bowl, whisk together flour, sugar, baking powder, and salt.
3. In another bowl, mix milk, cannabis-infused vegetable oil, egg, and vanilla extract.
4. Add the wet ingredients to the dry ingredients and stir until just combined.
5. Fold in chocolate chips.
6. Divide the batter evenly among the muffin cups.
7. Bake for 18-20 minutes or until a toothpick inserted comes out clean.

8. Allow to cool before serving.

9. Enjoy your cannabis-infused chocolate chip muffins!

Nutritional Information (per serving):

- Calories: 350
- Protein: 6g
- Carbohydrates: 45g
- Fat: 15g
- Fiber: 2g

Drinks

31. Lemon Cannabis Iced Tea

Ingredients for 4:

- 4 cups black tea, brewed and cooled

- 1/2 cup cannabis-infused simple syrup

- 1 lemon, sliced

- Ice cubes

Preparation Time: 10 minutes
Total Time: 10 minutes

Procedure:

1. In a pitcher, combine brewed black tea and cannabis-infused simple syrup.

2. Stir well to mix.

3. Add lemon slices to the pitcher.

4. Refrigerate until chilled.

5. Serve over ice and enjoy your cannabis-infused lemon iced tea!

Nutritional Information (per serving):

- Calories: 50

- Protein: 0g

- Carbohydrates: 15g

- Fat: 0g

- Fiber: 0g

32. Cannabis infused Fruit Smoothie

Ingredients for 4:

- 2 cups mixed frozen fruits (berries, mango, pineapple)
- 1 banana
- 1 cup cannabis-infused coconut water
- 1/2 cup Greek yogurt
- Honey to taste

Preparation Time: 10 minutes
Total Time: 10 minutes

Procedure:

1. In a blender, combine mixed frozen fruits, banana, cannabis-infused coconut water, and Greek yogurt.
2. Blend until smooth.
3. Sweeten with honey to taste.
4. Pour into glasses and enjoy your cannabis-infused fruit smoothie!

Nutritional Information (per serving):

- Calories: 150
- Protein: 3g
- Carbohydrates: 35g
- Fat: 1g
- Fiber: 5g

33. Cannabis Flavored Milk

Ingredients for 4:

- 4 cups milk
- 1/2 cup cannabis-infused chocolate syrup (or other flavor)
- Whipped cream for topping (optional)

Preparation Time: 5 minutes
Total Time: 5 minutes

Procedure:

1. In a pitcher, combine milk and cannabis-infused chocolate syrup.
2. Stir well to mix.
3. Pour into glasses.
4. Top with whipped cream if desired.
5. Enjoy your cannabis-infused flavored milk!

Nutritional Information (per serving):

- Calories: 120
- Protein: 8g
- Carbohydrates: 20g
- Fat: 2.5g
- Fiber: 0g

Cocktails

34. Cannabis Margarita

Ingredients for 4:

- 1 cup tequila
- 1/2 cup triple sec
- 1/2 cup lime juice
- 1/4 cup cannabis-infused simple syrup
- Salt for rimming glasses
- Lime wedges for garnish

Preparation Time: 10 minutes
Total Time: 10 minutes

Procedure:

1. Rim glasses with salt.
2. In a shaker, combine tequila, triple sec, lime juice, and cannabis-infused simple syrup.
3. Shake well.
4. Strain into prepared glasses over ice.
5. Garnish with lime wedges.
6. Sip and enjoy your cannabis-infused margarita!

Nutritional Information (per serving):

- Calories: 200
- Protein: 0g
- Carbohydrates: 15g
- Fat: 0g
- Fiber: 0g

35. Minty Cannabis Mojito

Ingredients for 4:

- 1 cup white rum
- 1/2 cup fresh lime juice
- 1/4 cup cannabis-infused simple syrup
- 1 cup mint leaves
- Club soda
- Lime wedges for garnish

Preparation Time: 10 minutes
Total Time: 10 minutes

Procedure:

1. In a pitcher, muddle mint leaves with lime juice and cannabis-infused simple syrup.
2. Add white rum and stir.
3. Fill glasses with ice.
4. Pour the mint and rum mixture over the ice.
5. Top with club soda.
6. Garnish with lime wedges.
7. Enjoy your cannabis-infused mojito!

Nutritional Information (per serving):

- Calories: 150
- Protein: 0g
- Carbohydrates: 15g
- Fat: 0g
- Fiber: 0g

36. Passion Fruit Cannabis Punch

Ingredients for 4:

- 1 cup passion fruit juice
- 1/2 cup pineapple juice
- 1/4 cup cannabis-infused simple syrup
- 1 cup orange juice
- 1 cup soda water
- Orange slices for garnish

Preparation Time: 10 minutes
Total Time: 10 minutes

Procedure:

1. In a pitcher, combine passion fruit juice, pineapple juice, cannabis-infused simple syrup, and orange juice.
2. Stir well.
3. Add soda water and stir again.
4. Serve over ice.
5. Garnish with orange slices.
6. Enjoy your cannabis-infused passion fruit punch!

Nutritional Information (per serving):

- Calories: 100
- Protein: 1g
- Carbohydrates: 25g
- Fat: 0g
- Fiber: 1g

Indulge in these delightful cannabis-infused desserts and beverages responsibly!

Ice creams and Sorbets

37. Cannabis Vanilla Ice Cream

Ingredients for 4:

- 2 cups heavy cream
- 1 cup whole milk
- 3/4 cup granulated sugar
- 1 tablespoon vanilla extract
- 1/4 cup cannabis-infused cream

Preparation Time: 15 minutes
Churn Time: 30 minutes
Freeze Time: 4 hours

Procedure:

1. In a bowl, whisk together heavy cream, whole milk, sugar, vanilla extract, and cannabis-infused cream until sugar is dissolved.
2. Pour the mixture into an ice cream maker and churn according to the manufacturer's instructions.
3. Transfer the churned ice cream to a lidded container and freeze for at least 4 hours.
4. Scoop and enjoy your cannabis-infused vanilla ice cream!

Nutritional Information (per serving):

- Calories: 350
- Protein: 3g
- Carbohydrates: 25g
- Fat: 27g
- Fiber: 0g

38. Cannabis Lemon Sorbet

Ingredients for 4:

- 1 cup water
- 1 cup granulated sugar
- 1 cup fresh lemon juice
- 1 tablespoon lemon zest
- 1/4 cup cannabis-infused simple syrup

Preparation Time: 10 minutes
Chill Time: 4 hours
Total Time: 4 hours 10 minutes

Procedure:

1. In a saucepan, combine water and sugar. Heat over medium until sugar is dissolved.

2. Remove from heat and let it cool to room temperature.

3. Stir in fresh lemon juice, lemon zest, and cannabis-infused simple syrup.

4. Pour the mixture into an ice cream maker and churn according to the manufacturer's instructions.

5. Transfer the churned sorbet to a lidded container and freeze for at least 4 hours.

6. Scoop and enjoy your cannabis-infused lemon sorbet!

Nutritional Information (per serving):

- Calories: 150
- Protein: 0g
- Carbohydrates: 40g
- Fat: 0g
- Fiber: 0g

39. Cannabis Berry Popsicle

Ingredients for 4:

- 1 cup mixed berries (strawberries, blueberries, raspberries)
- 1/4 cup cannabis-infused simple syrup
- 1 cup coconut water

Preparation Time: 10 minutes
Freeze Time: 4 hours
Total Time: 4 hours 10 minutes

Procedure:

1. Blend mixed berries and cannabis-infused simple syrup until smooth.
2. Pour the berry mixture into popsicle molds, filling each mold about halfway.
3. Add coconut water to the molds, leaving a little space at the top.
4. Insert popsicle sticks and freeze for at least 4 hours.
5. Unmold and enjoy your cannabis-infused berry popsicles!

Nutritional Information (per serving):

- Calories: 50
- Protein: 0g
- Carbohydrates: 15g
- Fat: 0g
- Fiber: 3g

Street Food

40. Cannabis Cheesy Pretzel with Sauce

Ingredients for 4:

- 1 lb pizza dough
- 1/4 cup cannabis-infused butter, melted
- 1/2 cup shredded cheddar cheese
- Salt for sprinkling
- 1/4 cup cannabis-infused cheese sauce (for dipping)

Preparation Time: 15 minutes
Bake Time: 15 minutes
Total Time: 30 minutes

Procedure:

1. Preheat the oven to 475°F (245°C).
2. Roll out the pizza dough and cut into strips.
3. Twist each strip and place on a baking sheet.
4. Brush with melted cannabis-infused butter and sprinkle with shredded cheddar cheese and salt.
5. Bake for 12-15 minutes or until golden.
6. Serve with cannabis-infused cheese sauce for dipping.
7. Enjoy your cannabis-infused cheesy pretzel!

Nutritional Information (per serving):

- Calories: 300
- Protein: 8g
- Carbohydrates: 40g
- Fat: 15g
- Fiber: 2g

41. Cannabis Guacamole Nachos

Ingredients for 4:

- 1 bag tortilla chips
- 1 cup shredded cheddar cheese
- 1 cup cannabis-infused black beans, drained and rinsed
- 1 cup diced tomatoes
- 1/2 cup sliced jalapeños
- 1/2 cup cannabis-infused guacamole

Preparation Time: 10 minutes
Bake Time: 10 minutes
Total Time: 20 minutes

Procedure:

1. Preheat the oven to 375°F (190°C).
2. Arrange tortilla chips on a baking sheet.
3. Sprinkle shredded cheddar cheese over the chips.
4. Top with cannabis-infused black beans, diced tomatoes, and sliced jalapeños.
5. Bake for 8-10 minutes or until cheese is melted.
6. Remove from the oven and drizzle with cannabis-infused guacamole.
7. Serve your cannabis-infused nachos and enjoy!

Nutritional Information (per serving):

- Calories: 400
- Protein: 8g
- Carbohydrates: 30g
- Fat: 25g
- Fiber: 5g

42. Cannabis Caramelized Onion Hot Dog

Ingredients for 4:

- 4 hot dog buns
- 4 cannabis-infused beef hot dogs
- 1 cup caramelized onions
- 1/2 cup cannabis-infused mustard
- 1/4 cup chopped fresh parsley

Preparation Time: 15 minutes
Total Time: 15 minutes

Procedure:

1. Grill or heat the cannabis-infused beef hot dogs according to package instructions.
2. Place each hot dog in a bun.
3. Top with caramelized onions, cannabis-infused mustard, and chopped fresh parsley.
4. Serve your cannabis-infused caramelized onion hot dogs and enjoy!

Nutritional Information (per serving):

- Calories: 350
- Protein: 10g
- Carbohydrates: 30g
- Fat: 20g
- Fiber: 2g

Light Dishes

43. Cannabis Quinoa and Avocado Salad with Dressing

Ingredients for 4:

- 1 cup quinoa, cooked and cooled
- 1 avocado, diced
- 1 cup cherry tomatoes, halved
- 1/4 cup red onion, finely chopped
- 1/4 cup cannabis-infused olive oil
- 2 tablespoons balsamic vinegar
- Salt and pepper to taste
- Fresh basil for garnish

Preparation Time: 15 minutes
Total Time: 15 minutes

Procedure:

1. In a large bowl, combine cooked quinoa, diced avocado, cherry tomatoes, and chopped red onion.
2. In a small bowl, whisk together cannabis-infused olive oil and balsamic vinegar.
3. Drizzle the dressing over the quinoa mixture and toss gently.
4. Season with salt and pepper to taste.
5. Garnish with fresh basil.
6. Serve your cannabis-infused quinoa and avocado salad!

Nutritional Information (per serving):

- Calories: 300
- Protein: 6g
- Carbohydrates: 30g
- Fat: 18g
- Fiber: 6g

44. Cannabis Sushi with Soy Sauce
Ingredients for 4:

- 2 cups sushi rice, cooked and seasoned
- Nori sheets
- Assorted sushi fillings (avocado, cucumber, smoked salmon)
- Cannabis-infused soy sauce for dipping
- Pickled ginger and wasabi for serving

Preparation Time: 30 minutes
Total Time: 30 minutes

Procedure:

1. Place a nori sheet on a bamboo sushi mat.
2. Spread a thin layer of sushi rice over the nori, leaving a border at the top.
3. Add your choice of sushi fillings along the center.
4. Roll the sushi tightly using the bamboo mat.
5. Slice the sushi roll into bite-sized pieces.
6. Serve with cannabis-infused soy sauce, pickled ginger, and wasabi.
7. Enjoy your cannabis-infused sushi!

Nutritional Information (per serving):

- Calories: 250
- Protein: 5g
- Carbohydrates: 50g
- Fat: 2g
- Fiber: 3g

45. Cannabis Chicken Wrap with Sauce

Ingredients for 4:

- 4 large whole wheat tortillas
- 2 cups cooked and shredded chicken
- 1 cup mixed greens
- 1 cup cherry tomatoes, halved
- 1/2 cup feta cheese, crumbled
- 1/4 cup cannabis-infused dressing
- Salt and pepper to taste

Preparation Time: 15 minutes
Total Time: 15 minutes

Procedure:

1. In each tortilla, layer shredded chicken, mixed greens, cherry tomatoes, and crumbled feta cheese.
2. Drizzle cannabis-infused dressing over the fillings.
3. Season with salt and pepper to taste.
4. Fold in the sides of the tortilla and roll it up tightly.
5. Slice in half and serve your cannabis-infused chicken wrap!

Nutritional Information (per serving):

- Calories: 400
- Protein: 20g
- Carbohydrates: 30g
- Fat: 20g
- Fiber: 5g

Explore these flavorful cannabis-infused treats with a touch of creativity and a dash of excitement!

Mediterranean Cuisine

46. Cannabis Hummus with Pita

Ingredients for 4:

- 2 cans (15 oz each) chickpeas, drained and rinsed
- 1/2 cup cannabis-infused olive oil
- 1/4 cup tahini
- 2 cloves garlic, minced
- 1 teaspoon ground cumin
- Juice of 1 lemon
- Salt and pepper to taste
- Pitta bread for serving

Preparation Time: 10 minutes
Total Time: 10 minutes

Procedure:

1. In a food processor, combine chickpeas, cannabis-infused olive oil, tahini, minced garlic, ground cumin, and lemon juice.
2. Blend until smooth, adding more olive oil if needed.
3. Season with salt and pepper to taste.
4. Serve the cannabis-infused hummus with pitta bread.
5. Enjoy your Mediterranean-inspired cannabis-infused hummus!

Nutritional Information (per serving):

- Calories: 300
- Protein: 8g
- Carbohydrates: 20g
- Fat: 22g
- Fiber: 5g

47. Cannabis Eggplant Parmesan

Ingredients for 4:

- 2 large eggplants, sliced
- 1 cup cannabis-infused marinara sauce
- 1 cup breadcrumbs
- 1/2 cup grated Parmesan cheese
- 1 cup shredded mozzarella cheese
- Fresh basil for garnish

Preparation Time: 20 minutes
Bake Time: 30 minutes
Total Time: 50 minutes

Procedure:

1. Preheat the oven to 375°F (190°C).
2. Dip eggplant slices in cannabis-infused marinara sauce, then coat with a mixture of breadcrumbs and Parmesan cheese.
3. Arrange the coated eggplant slices in a baking dish.
4. Bake for 30 minutes or until golden and crispy.
5. Sprinkle shredded mozzarella cheese over the top and bake until melted.
6. Garnish with fresh basil.
7. Serve your cannabis-infused eggplant Parmesan and savor the flavors!

Nutritional Information (per serving):

- Calories: 350
- Protein: 15g
- Carbohydrates: 30g
- Fat: 18g
- Fiber: 8g

48. Cannabis Asparagus Risotto

Ingredients for 4:

- 2 cups Arborio rice
- 1 bunch asparagus, trimmed and sliced
- 1/2 cup dry white wine
- 4 cups vegetable broth, heated
- 1/2 cup grated Parmesan cheese
- 1/4 cup cannabis-infused olive oil
- Salt and pepper to taste

Preparation Time: 30 minutes
Total Time: 30 minutes

Procedure:

1. In a large pan, sauté Arborio rice in cannabis-infused olive oil until translucent.
2. Add sliced asparagus and cook for 2-3 minutes.
3. Pour in the dry white wine and stir until absorbed.
4. Gradually add hot vegetable broth, one ladle at a time, stirring constantly until rice is creamy and cooked.
5. Stir in grated Parmesan cheese.
6. Season with salt and pepper to taste.
7. Serve your cannabis-infused asparagus risotto and enjoy the Mediterranean flavors!

Nutritional Information (per serving):

- Calories: 400
- Protein: 8g
- Carbohydrates: 60g
- Fat: 12g
- Fiber: 4g

Vegan Dishes

49. Cannabis Chickpea Burger

Ingredients for 4:

- 2 cans (15 oz each) chickpeas, drained and rinsed
- 1/2 cup breadcrumbs
- 1/4 cup finely chopped red onion
- 1/4 cup chopped fresh parsley
- 1 teaspoon ground cumin
- 1/2 teaspoon smoked paprika
- Salt and pepper to taste
- Burger buns and toppings

Preparation Time: 15 minutes
Cook Time: 10 minutes
Total Time: 25 minutes

Procedure:

1. In a food processor, combine chickpeas, breadcrumbs, red onion, fresh parsley, ground cumin, smoked paprika, salt, and pepper.
2. Pulse until the mixture comes together.
3. Form the mixture into burger patties.
4. Cook on a grill or stovetop until golden on both sides.
5. Serve the cannabis-infused chickpea burgers on buns with your favorite toppings.
6. Enjoy a vegan delight with a cannabis twist!

Nutritional Information (per serving):

- Calories: 300
- Protein: 12g
- Carbohydrates: 50g
- Fat: 6g
- Fiber: 10g

50. Cannabis Vegetable Couscous
Ingredients for 4:

- 1 cup couscous
- 2 cups vegetable broth, heated
- 1 cup cherry tomatoes, halved
- 1 cup cucumber, diced
- 1/2 cup cannabis-infused olive oil
- 1/4 cup fresh mint, chopped
- Salt and pepper to taste

Preparation Time: 15 minutes
Total Time: 15 minutes

Procedure:

1. Place couscous in a bowl and pour hot vegetable broth over it.
2. Cover and let it sit for 5 minutes until the couscous absorbs the broth.
3. Fluff the couscous with a fork.
4. Add cherry tomatoes, diced cucumber, cannabis-infused olive oil, and chopped fresh mint.
5. Season with salt and pepper to taste.
6. Toss gently and serve your cannabis-infused vegetable couscous!
7. Enjoy the vegan goodness with a touch of cannabis!

Nutritional Information (per serving):

- Calories: 350
- Protein: 8g
- Carbohydrates: 50g
- Fat: 15g
- Fiber: 6g

51. Cannabis Tofu Curry

Ingredients for 4:

- 1 block firm tofu, cubed
- 1 cup broccoli florets
- 1 cup carrot slices
- 1 cup snow peas
- 1 can (14 oz) coconut milk
- 2 tablespoons cannabis-infused red curry paste
- 1 tablespoon soy sauce
- 1 tablespoon maple syrup
- Cooked rice for serving

Preparation Time: 20 minutes
Cook Time: 20 minutes
Total Time: 40 minutes

Procedure:

1. In a pan, sauté cubed tofu until golden.
2. Add broccoli, carrot slices, and snow peas.
3. Stir in cannabis-infused red curry paste, soy sauce, and maple syrup.
4. Pour in coconut milk and simmer until vegetables are tender.
5. Serve the cannabis-infused tofu curry over cooked rice.
6. Enjoy a flavorful vegan meal with a touch of cannabis!

Nutritional Information (per serving):

- Calories: 400
- Protein: 15g
- Carbohydrates: 30g
- Fat: 25g
- Fiber: 8g

Breakfast Dishes

52. Cannabis Pancakes with Maple Syrup
Ingredients for 4:

- 2 cups pancake mix
- 1 cup milk
- 1 egg
- 1/4 cup cannabis-infused maple syrup
- Fresh berries for topping

Preparation Time: 15 minutes
Cook Time: 10 minutes
Total Time: 25 minutes

Procedure:

1. In a bowl, whisk together pancake mix, milk, and egg until smooth.
2. Heat a griddle or pan over medium heat.
3. Pour pancake batter onto the griddle to form pancakes.
4. Cook until bubbles form on the surface, then flip and cook the other side.
5. Drizzle cannabis-infused maple syrup over the pancakes.
6. Top with fresh berries and enjoy your cannabis-infused pancakes!

Nutritional Information (per serving):

- Calories: 300
- Protein: 8g
- Carbohydrates: 50g
- Fat: 8g
- Fiber: 2g

53. Cannabis Smoothie Bowl

Ingredients for 4:

- 2 cups frozen mixed berries

- 1 frozen banana

- 1 cup coconut milk

- 1/4 cup cannabis-infused granola

- Fresh fruit and nuts for topping

Preparation Time: 10 minutes
Total Time: 10 minutes

Procedure:

1. Blend frozen mixed berries, frozen banana, and coconut milk until smooth.

2. Pour the smoothie into bowls.

3. Top with cannabis-infused granola, fresh fruit, and nuts.

4. Enjoy a refreshing cannabis-infused smoothie bowl for breakfast!

Nutritional Information (per serving):

- Calories: 250

- Protein: 5g

- Carbohydrates: 40g

- Fat: 10g

- Fiber: 6g

54. Apple Cannabis Porridge

Ingredients for 4:

- 1 cup rolled oats
- 2 cups milk
- 1 apple, grated
- 1/4 cup cannabis-infused honey
- Cinnamon for sprinkling

Preparation Time: 15 minutes
Cook Time: 10 minutes
Total Time: 25 minutes

Procedure:

1. In a saucepan, combine rolled oats and milk.
2. Cook over medium heat, stirring until oats are tender.
3. Stir in grated apple and cannabis-infused honey.
4. Continue cooking until the porridge reaches your desired consistency.
5. Sprinkle with cinnamon before serving.
6. Enjoy a warm and comforting cannabis-infused apple porridge!

Nutritional Information (per serving):

- Calories: 300
- Protein: 8g
- Carbohydrates: 50g
- Fat: 6g
- Fiber: 8g

Autumn Dishes

55. Cannabis Stuffed Pumpkin

Ingredients for 4:

- 1 small sugar pumpkin
- 2 cups cooked quinoa
- 1 cup cannabis-infused black beans, drained and rinsed
- 1 cup diced vegetables (bell peppers, onions, corn)
- 1/2 cup shredded cheddar cheese
- 1/4 cup cannabis-infused olive oil
- Salt and pepper to taste

Preparation Time: 20 minutes
Bake Time: 40 minutes
Total Time: 1 hour

Procedure:

1. Preheat the oven to 375°F (190°C).
2. Cut the top off the pumpkin and remove seeds and pulp.
3. In a bowl, combine cooked quinoa, cannabis-infused black beans, diced vegetables, shredded cheddar cheese, and cannabis-infused olive oil.
4. Season with salt and pepper to taste.
5. Stuff the pumpkin with the quinoa mixture.
6. Place the pumpkin on a baking sheet and bake for 40 minutes or until the pumpkin is tender.
7. Slice and serve your cannabis-infused stuffed pumpkin!

Nutritional Information (per serving):

- Calories: 350
- Protein: 10g
- Carbohydrates: 40g
- Fat: 18g
- Fiber: 8g

56. Cannabis Apple Cake

Ingredients for 4:

- 2 cups diced apples
- 2 cups all-purpose flour
- 1 cup granulated sugar
- 1/2 cup cannabis-infused butter, melted
- 2 eggs
- 1 teaspoon vanilla extract
- 1 teaspoon ground cinnamon
- 1/2 teaspoon baking powder
- 1/2 teaspoon baking soda
- 1/4 teaspoon salt

Preparation Time: 15 minutes
Bake Time: 45 minutes
Total Time: 1 hour

Procedure:

1. Preheat the oven to 350°F (175°C).
2. In a bowl, mix diced apples with sugar and let it sit for 10 minutes.
3. In another bowl, whisk together flour, cannabis-infused butter, eggs, vanilla extract, ground cinnamon, baking powder, baking soda, and salt.
4. Fold in the apple mixture.
5. Pour the batter into a greased baking pan.
6. Bake for 45 minutes or until a toothpick comes out clean.
7. Allow to cool before slicing and serving your cannabis-infused apple cake!

Nutritional Information (per serving):

- Calories: 400
- Protein: 5g
- Carbohydrates: 60g
- Fat: 18g
- Fiber: 3g

57. Cannabis Porcini Mushroom Risotto

Ingredients for 4:

- 2 cups Arborio rice
- 1 cup dried porcini mushrooms, rehydrated
- 1/2 cup white wine
- 1/4 cup cannabis-infused olive oil
- 1 onion, finely chopped
- 2 cloves garlic, minced
- 4 cups vegetable broth, warm
- 1/2 cup grated Parmesan cheese
- Salt and pepper to taste

Preparation Time: 30 minutes
Cook Time: 25 minutes
Total Time: 55 minutes

Procedure:

1. In a skillet, heat cannabis-infused olive oil and sauté onions until translucent.
2. Add garlic and Arborio rice, stirring until the rice is lightly toasted.
3. Pour in the white wine and cook until it's mostly absorbed.
4. Begin adding warm vegetable broth, one ladle at a time, stirring frequently until absorbed.
5. Continue this process until the rice is creamy and cooked to al dente.
6. Stir in rehydrated porcini mushrooms and grated Parmesan cheese.
7. Season with salt and pepper to taste.

8. Serve your cannabis-infused porcini mushroom risotto hot!

Nutritional Information (per serving):

- Calories: 400
- Protein: 10g
- Carbohydrates: 70g
- Fat: 10g
- Fiber: 5g

Winter Dishes

58. Cannabis Hot Chocolate

Ingredients for 4:

- 4 cups milk
- 1/2 cup cannabis-infused chocolate chips
- 1/4 cup cocoa powder
- 1/4 cup sugar
- 1 teaspoon vanilla extract
- Whipped cream and chocolate shavings for garnish

Preparation Time: 10 minutes
Total Time: 10 minutes

Procedure:

1. In a saucepan, heat milk until warm but not boiling.
2. Whisk in cannabis-infused chocolate chips, cocoa powder, sugar, and vanilla extract.
3. Continue whisking until the chocolate chips are melted and the mixture is smooth.
4. Pour into mugs and top with whipped cream and chocolate shavings.
5. Enjoy your cannabis-infused hot chocolate!

Nutritional Information (per serving):

- Calories: 250
- Protein: 8g
- Carbohydrates: 30g
- Fat: 12g
- Fiber: 3g

59. Cannabis Roast Chicken with Potatoes

Ingredients for 4:

- 1 whole chicken (about 4 lbs)
- 1/4 cup cannabis-infused olive oil
- 2 teaspoons dried thyme
- 1 teaspoon paprika
- 1 teaspoon garlic powder
- Salt and pepper to taste
- 1 lb baby potatoes, halved

Preparation Time: 20 minutes
Roast Time: 1 hour 30 minutes
Total Time: 1 hour 50 minutes

Procedure:

1. Preheat the oven to 375°F (190°C).
2. Rub the chicken with cannabis-infused olive oil, dried thyme, paprika, garlic powder, salt, and pepper.
3. Place the seasoned chicken in a roasting pan.
4. Toss the halved baby potatoes in any remaining cannabis-infused olive oil and seasonings.
5. Arrange the potatoes around the chicken in the roasting pan.
6. Roast for 1 hour and 30 minutes or until the chicken is cooked through.
7. Let it rest before carving.
8. Serve your cannabis-infused roast chicken with potatoes!

Nutritional Information (per serving):

- Calories: 500
- Protein: 30g
- Carbohydrates: 20g
- Fat: 35g
- Fiber: 3g

60. Cannabis Lentil Soup

Ingredients for 4:

- 1 cup dry green lentils, rinsed

- 1 onion, chopped

- 2 carrots, diced

- 2 celery stalks, chopped

- 3 cloves garlic, minced

- 6 cups vegetable broth

- 1 can (14 oz) diced tomatoes

- 1 teaspoon ground cumin

- 1/2 teaspoon smoked paprika

- Salt and pepper to taste

- Fresh parsley for garnish

Preparation Time: 15 minutes
Cook Time: 40 minutes
Total Time: 55 minutes

Procedure:

1. In a large pot, combine dry green lentils, chopped onion, diced carrots, chopped celery, minced garlic, vegetable broth, diced tomatoes, ground cumin, and smoked paprika.

2. Bring to a boil, then reduce heat and simmer for 40 minutes or until lentils are tender.

3. Season with salt and pepper to taste.

4. Garnish with fresh parsley.

5. Serve your cannabis-infused lentil soup hot!

Nutritional Information (per serving):

- Calories: 300
- Protein: 18g
- Carbohydrates: 50g
- Fat: 5g
- Fiber: 15g

Spring Dishes

61. Cannabis Strawberry and Spinach Salad with Balsamic

Ingredients for 4:

- 4 cups fresh spinach leaves
- 2 cups sliced strawberries
- 1/2 cup crumbled feta cheese
- 1/4 cup cannabis-infused balsamic vinaigrette
- 1/4 cup candied pecans
- Salt and pepper to taste

Preparation Time: 15 minutes
Total Time: 15 minutes

Procedure:

1. In a large bowl, combine fresh spinach leaves, sliced strawberries, and crumbled feta cheese.
2. Drizzle cannabis-infused balsamic vinaigrette over the salad and toss gently.
3. Top with candied pecans.
4. Season with salt and pepper to taste.
5. Serve your cannabis-infused strawberry and spinach salad!

Nutritional Information (per serving):

- Calories: 200
- Protein: 5g
- Carbohydrates: 20g
- Fat: 12g
- Fiber: 5g

62. Cannabis Asparagus Risotto

Ingredients for 4:

- 2 cups Arborio rice
- 1 bunch asparagus, trimmed and cut into bite-sized pieces
- 1/2 cup dry white wine
- 1/4 cup cannabis-infused olive oil
- 1 onion, finely chopped
- 2 cloves garlic, minced
- 4 cups vegetable broth, warm
- 1/2 cup grated Parmesan cheese
- Salt and pepper to taste

Preparation Time: 30 minutes
Cook Time: 25 minutes
Total Time: 55 minutes

Procedure:

1. In a skillet, heat cannabis-infused olive oil and sauté onions until translucent.
2. Add garlic and Arborio rice, stirring until the rice is lightly toasted.
3. Pour in the white wine and cook until it's mostly absorbed.
4. Begin adding warm vegetable broth, one ladle at a time, stirring frequently until absorbed.
5. Continue this process until the rice is creamy and cooked to al dente.
6. Stir in the asparagus pieces and grated Parmesan cheese.
7. Season with salt and pepper to taste.
8. Serve your cannabis-infused asparagus risotto hot!

Nutritional Information (per serving):

- Calories: 400
- Protein: 10g
- Carbohydrates: 70g
- Fat: 10g
- Fiber: 5g

63. Cannabis Spring Frittata

Ingredients for 4:

- 6 large eggs
- 1/2 cup milk
- 1 cup diced bell peppers (assorted colors)
- 1 cup cherry tomatoes, halved
- 1/2 cup feta cheese, crumbled
- 1/4 cup cannabis-infused olive oil
- Salt and pepper to taste
- Fresh herbs for garnish

Preparation Time: 15 minutes
Cook Time: 20 minutes
Total Time: 35 minutes

Procedure:

1. Preheat the oven to 375°F (190°C).
2. In a bowl, whisk together eggs and milk.
3. Stir in diced bell peppers, cherry tomatoes, and crumbled feta cheese.
4. In an oven-safe skillet, heat cannabis-infused olive oil over medium heat.
5. Pour the egg mixture into the skillet.
6. Cook for 3-5 minutes, stirring occasionally.
7. Transfer the skillet to the preheated oven and bake for 15-20 minutes or until the frittata is set.
8. Garnish with fresh herbs.
9. Slice and serve your cannabis-infused spring frittata!

Nutritional Information (per serving):

- Calories: 300
- Protein: 15g
- Carbohydrates: 10g
- Fat: 20g
- Fiber: 3g

Summer Dishes

64. Cannabis Greek Salad with Feta

Ingredients for 4:

- 4 cups chopped romaine lettuce
- 1 cucumber, diced
- 1 cup cherry tomatoes, halved
- 1/2 cup red onion, thinly sliced
- 1/2 cup crumbled feta cheese
- 1/4 cup cannabis-infused Greek dressing
- Kalamata olives for garnish
- Salt and pepper to taste

Preparation Time: 15 minutes
Total Time: 15 minutes

Procedure:

1. In a large bowl, combine chopped romaine lettuce, diced cucumber, cherry tomatoes, red onion, and crumbled feta cheese.
2. Drizzle cannabis-infused Greek dressing over the salad and toss gently.
3. Garnish with Kalamata olives.
4. Season with salt and pepper to taste.
5. Serve your cannabis-infused Greek salad!

Nutritional Information (per serving):

- Calories: 250
- Protein: 8g
- Carbohydrates: 15g
- Fat: 18g
- Fiber: 5g

65. Cannabis Barbecue Pork with Barbecue Sauce

Ingredients for 4:

- 4 pork chops
- 1 cup cannabis-infused barbecue sauce
- 1 teaspoon smoked paprika
- 1 teaspoon garlic powder
- Salt and pepper to taste

Preparation Time: 10 minutes
Grill Time: 20 minutes
Total Time: 30 minutes

Procedure:

1. Preheat the grill to medium-high heat.
2. Season pork chops with smoked paprika, garlic powder, salt, and pepper.
3. Grill the pork chops for about 10 minutes per side or until they reach the desired doneness.
4. Brush cannabis-infused barbecue sauce over the pork chops during the last few minutes of grilling.
5. Serve your cannabis-infused barbecue pork hot off the grill!

Nutritional Information (per serving):

- Calories: 400
- Protein: 25g
- Carbohydrates: 30g
- Fat: 18g
- Fiber: 2g

66. Cannabis Grilled Shrimp
Ingredients for 4:

- 1 lb large shrimp, peeled and deveined
- 1/4 cup cannabis-infused olive oil
- 2 cloves garlic, minced
- 1 teaspoon smoked paprika
- 1/2 teaspoon red pepper flakes
- 1 lemon, juiced
- Fresh parsley for garnish
- Salt and pepper to taste

Preparation Time: 15 minutes
Grill Time: 5 minutes
Total Time: 20 minutes

Procedure:

1. In a bowl, combine cannabis-infused olive oil, minced garlic, smoked paprika, red pepper flakes, lemon juice, salt, and pepper.
2. Add the peeled and deveined shrimp to the marinade, tossing to coat evenly.
3. Preheat the grill to medium-high heat.
4. Thread shrimp onto skewers.
5. Grill the shrimp for about 2-3 minutes per side or until they are opaque.
6. Garnish with fresh parsley.
7. Serve your cannabis-infused grilled shrimp hot off the grill!

Nutritional Information (per serving):

- Calories: 200
- Protein: 20g
- Carbohydrates: 2g
- Fat: 12g
- Fiber: 1g

Thanks for buying:

STEP 1: Consider posting a quick review on Amazon, every review counts and is deeply appreciated

STEP 2: scan the QR CODE and download the bonus recipes: Marijuana-infused Body Hydrating Cream and Cannabis-infused Nourishing Hair Oil

If the Qr code isn't working, write an email to: sse047748@gmail.com